STOP AGING
AGING

or

Slow the Process

William Campbell Douglass, MD

D1329413

Second Opinion Publishing

ISBN 1-885236-02-6

Cover design by Elizabeth Bame

Additional copies of this book may be purchased from Second Opinion Publishing for $8.95. Second Opinion Publishing also publishes Dr. Douglass's monthly "contrary opinion" medical newsletter, *Second Opinion*. An introductory subscription to *Second Opinion* is $49 for 1 year, $89 for 2 years. To subscribe or obtain more information regarding Second Opinion products, please call or write:

Second Opinion Publishing, Inc.
Post Office Box 467939
Atlanta, Georgia 31146-7939
800-728-2288 or 404-399-5617

Contents

Other Books by
William Campbell Douglass, MD

*AIDS: Why It's Much Worse Than
They're Telling Us and How To Protect Yourself and
Your Loved Ones*

Bad Medicine

Eat Your Cholesterol

Dangerous (Legal) Drugs

Hydrogen Peroxide: Medical Miracle

Into the Light

The Milk Book

Prostate Problems: Safe, Simple, Effective Relief

Introduction

What is Exercise With Oxygen Therapy?

EWOT — it sounds like the counter girl at the Greasy Spoon calling out orders to the frantic cook in the smoke-filled kitchen: "Give us a hamburger — EWOT" — everything without the tomato. But it's a lot more important than that. An example:

Andy J. was a 75 year old retired theatrical agent. He was depressed and so debilitated, mentally and physically, that he couldn't put one foot in front of the other without sitting down to rest. He and Theresa, a former, well-known professional classic dancer, had been married for 50 years. Andy had a seemingly illimitable sexual appetite and Theresa was not far behind in the enjoyment of the Oldest Sport.

Around the age of 60, Andy's biological systems began to wane, and an important part of their life disappeared, almost overnight. At first, Theresa accused him of infidelity and of not loving her anymore. It was inconceivable that it could be anything else in a man who seemed to think of little but sex and sports.

Theresa brought Andy in for a "check up," but what she really wanted, and confessed privately after the exam, was her old vigorous animal Andy back. As I had suspected, he didn't have serious cardiovascular disease, his prostate was normal, and there really seemed to be no reason for his lack of energy and eclipsed sexual appetite except (and you never tell a patient this) old age.

I explained to them that Andy's problem was due to his inability to take up oxygen efficiently, which was, in turn, caused by a deficiency of certain enzymes. I had just begun the study of a new treatment called Exercise With

Oxygen Therapy (EWOT) and suggested that we put him on the program, three times a week.

Two weeks after starting the treatment, I had a call from Theresa: "Doctor Douglass, I have a new problem. Can you turn the thermostat back down a little? You've over shot the mark and he thinks he's on his honeymoon!" She didn't *really* want any adjustments; that was just her way of saying thank you. When I next saw Andy, who was sensitive about his impotence and had never mentioned it to me, I asked him how things were going. He answered, "Fine, Doc; everything's fine." I then asked him if there had been any dramatic changes in his life and he replied: "Nope, I feel great; everything's fine."

Not everyone is going to have this dramatic a result. But with Andy I was afraid he would kill himself. Five years later, they were still smiling and usually holding hands.

In all my years of practice, I haven't seen anything so simple that can accomplish so much. I am convinced that EWOT can prolong useful and enjoyable life and you'll look as pink as a new-born baby!

The Benefits of Oxygen

The three basic "nutrients" without which planet earth could not exist as a home for living things are light, water, and oxygen. I am currently writing two special reports on water and the use of *externally applied* light for treating various ailments. But this report is on the use of oxygen in a way that is both simple and effective for the prevention of aging and improving your health. EWOT (pronounced ee-watt) stands for Exercise With Oxygen Therapy. This method of prolonging your life is so simple that it's hard to believe it could work, but it does and you can do it at home at a minimal cost.

The main reason for aging, as with our patient Andy J., is the failure of enzymatic systems that are responsible for your body's *uptake and utilization of oxygen*. When your cells don't get enough oxygen, they degenerate and die and so *you* degenerate and die. It's as simple as that.

The world-renown physicist Dr. Manfred von Ardenne made a very significant discovery that should have stimulated vigorous research in how to maintain oxygen utilization in the body. He is best known for his work on the construction of the atomic bomb for the Soviets, but his work on oxygen utilization has been largely ignored outside his own institute.

Von Ardenne discovered, after measuring the oxygen blood levels in thousands of volunteers, that stressing factors, such as physical or mental overstrain (death of a loved one), complete lack of exercise (absolute bed rest), intoxications, infections, operations (or even anxiety about a forthcoming operation), radiation and other high-energy types of medical therapy, cancer, immunizations, drugs (legitimate and illegitimate), smoking, trauma, and even "focal" infections such as a boil or abscessed tooth, *can cause a dramatic and serious decline in your ability to absorb oxygen into your blood.*

Human beings can take a lot of punishment, mentally and physically, so these frequent drops in your ability to utilize oxygen efficiently are not going to kill you immediately. You would have died a long time ago if that were true. But each oxygen deprivation can take it's toll, and if a few cells die here and there due to constant external (or internal) stress, it begins to add up. The end result is premature aging.

So if a simple system can be used that constantly provides the body with additional oxygen, these stress factors can be, to a certain extent, neutralized. With EWOT that system is easily available.

Exercising, while breathing oxygen, dramatically increases the amount of oxygen in the blood plasma, i.e., the portion of the blood outside the red and white cells. This can be easily determined by testing the blood oxygen level in the arteries or veins. Doctors will say that you can't increase the oxygen in your blood by breathing oxygen. But what they mean is that you can't increase the amount of oxygen *in your red blood cells*, which are responsible for transporting oxygen to the tissues. The reason the amount of oxygen in the red cells cannot be increased is because, under most circumstances, they are already 97 percent saturated with oxygen. So, they say, a three percent increase will make little difference and the red cells won't accept the extra oxygen, anyway.

While this is true, they ignore the role of oxygen in the plasma, the "juice" within which the red cells flow. The oxygen content of this fluid can be *dramatically* increased and thus oxygen will be "pushed" into the body's cells without the aid of the red cells. It's called the Law of Mass Action. If you build up the concentration of a certain component in a chemical mixture high enough, chemical combining will take place with other elements of the mixture that ordinarily wouldn't happen.

Most of the oxygen in the plasma under these high-saturation circumstances will be "wasted" in that it will not be absorbed by the cells which expect to be "fed" oxygen by the red cells. But if only one tenth of one percent of the oxygen gets through, and you offer your cells this extra "meal" every day, there will be an extensive increase in your total tissue oxygen level. The objective is to keep the oxygen level of your blood as close to optimum (100 points) as long as possible; ideally, for your entire life.

After 15 minutes of EWOT, there is a dramatic "pinking up" of a patient's skin. If this can be seen so easily by simple observation, then it is obvious that the tiny capillaries, vessels tinier than a strand of hair, are carrying extra oxygen to cells of the body. Presumably, although this is a little more difficult to prove, every organ (your brain, kidneys, heart, eyes, and even the tips of your toes) is being bathed in extra amounts of life-sustaining oxygen.

But You Said ...

Some may see a contradiction in this report and my long-standing admonition not to overdo the exercise craze by jogging yourself to death. The theory is that if you exercise vigorously, you will increase the oxygenation of the blood and hence your tissues. But this is not true. You can run ten miles and you will not increase the oxygen content of your blood. You will, in fact, temporarily *decrease* your blood oxygen as the body burns oxygen to cover the work load.

I definitely don't believe a sedentary lifestyle is healthy, either. In fact, very moderate exercise, as in walking, has again been confirmed as the best exercise. A recent article by Jane Brody of the *New York Times* reported on the findings of a University of Iowa study indicating that frequent walks reduced by half the likelihood of developing gastrointestinal hemorrhage. It is well-known that during exercise, blood is sent to the muscles to provide oxygen where it is immediately needed. And the blood is not "oxygen-enriched" – the longer you exercise, the less oxygen the blood contains. That's why you feel fatigued after heavy exercise.

What we are recommending is not strenuous

exercise, but exercise for a limited period of time, 15 minutes, in the presence of extra oxygen. *This will give you* "oxygen-rich blood."

Chapter 1

The Benefits Are Universal

Let me ask a question that is simple to answer: If doing simple exercise daily for 15 minutes while breathing oxygen through your nose would enable you to have an oxygen status *higher than the average 30-year-old*, would you be interested in such a treatment. Especially since it only costs pennies, is safe, and can be done in the privacy of your own home?

This technique is so simple that one

wonders why no one investigated it until 20 years ago. And, equally important, why no one has followed up on the original work by Dr. von Ardenne.

Dr. von Ardenne's research on the subject of oxygen therapy is quite detailed and impressive. By 1981, he had done more than *10,000 measurements* of blood oxygen in patients and had proven the remarkable reactivity of the body to an increase in blood oxygen. He demonstrated the effects of stress, both psychological and physical, in lowering the blood oxygen levels and thus contributing to disease and aging. He observed, for instance, a significant rise in blood oxygen in normal persons after three weeks of rest and relaxation in the mountains. This couldn't be due to getting more oxygen from the "mountain air" as there is *less* oxygen at higher altitudes. He concluded that the increase in oxygen was due to lessening of stress which opened the body's oxygen-producing capacity.

To give you a better idea of how effective EWOT can be for specific illnesses let's take a look at a few case studies:

Heart Failure

Patients with heart failure are uniformly helped with EWOT. In every case I have treated, the result was an increased exercise tolerance. Many could walk for blocks following therapy. Whereas before treatment they often couldn't walk out to the mailbox and back without taking a rest.

Mary K., a wealthy heiress of a New England timber fortune, was a wonderful lady who was very involved in our community. She was a vigorous campaigner for improving our city, both with funding and personal effort, and an implacable foe of crooked politicians. She was 80 and had suffered two attacks of pulmonary edema, a filling of the lungs with fluid due to heart failure. Her heart had swelled to twice its normal size ("cardiomegaly"), so her outlook was dim indeed. With pulmonary edema, the third attack is usually fatal.

Against her cardiologist's advice (he had not told her about the "three strikes and you're out" rule) she elected to take EWOT. She knew that the digitalis and Lasix were not going to prevent Strike Three. They hadn't prevented Strike Two, so why would you expect any base hits? Smart lady.

Because of her very weak heart, we started Mary on a program of very modified EWOT. While she was lying down and breathing oxygen, we had her hold small weights and flex her arms. As she grew stronger, we gradually increased the amount of exercise and the weight. We admonished her to be patient (not one of her outstanding virtues) and to write down her impressions of her progress, if any, on a daily basis. Within a month, she had a *book* and was regaling us, her friends, and her doctors on the wonders of EWOT. In three months, she was asking my opinion as to the advisability of a little plastic surgery! (I think she had Club Med on her mind.)

We managed to keep her focused on the welfare of the city and dogging the politicians. Her heart came down to a normal size and, eight years later, she had not had a another attack of pulmonary edema, but she *did* get the plastic surgery!

Alzheimer's

I have also treated two Alzheimer's patients with EWOT. It was very difficult because of their inability to focus on anything for very long. But with constant supervision and encouragement, they could be "hyper-oxygenated" with EWOT. Both of them showed considerable improvement, but the routine was exhausting the family and they finally, in both cases, gave up. As a result, I never had any conclusive evidence that EWOT was making a difference. Because of the difficulty of treating advanced cases, I think the only effective way will be to start them on EWOT while they're in the early stages. I doubt that Alzheimer's disease can be reversed with EWOT, but I think the progress of the disease can be arrested.

Emphysema

Emphysema, in some cases, will have a dramatic response. But the patient must continue the treatment indefinitely because, once EWOT is discontinued, he will deteriorate over a period of a few months.

Our most dramatic case of emphysema was a 75-year-old man, a retired automobile executive, who was wheeled into the office by his wife. He was blue around the lips and so short of breath that he could hardly talk. He had to sleep sitting up and was starving because he couldn't eat and breathe at the same time. He was six feet tall and weighed 140 pounds.

We had to be even more careful than with Mary K. because of his precarious lung condition. Over a period of six months, he improved enough to abandon his wheelchair and at the end of the first year went on a Caribbean cruise with his wife.

Stress

But the most dramatic results have been seen in those patients who are really stressed to the limit. According to Dr. von Ardenne, people who have experienced a recent divorce, the death of a loved one, the loss of a job, or some other financial assault have a uniformly low blood-oxygen level. Obviously, you can't cure the problem with oxygen, but the treatment is very effective in restoring the coping mentality that is needed to see them through.

One of our more poignant cases was a 45-year-old man whose daughter had committed suicide. He was so depressed and ridden with guilt he could hardly dress himself: What had he done? What *hadn't* he done? What *should* he have done?

He was literally crushing himself to death.

His frantic wife brought him in, against his will, asking us to do something. She had no faith or trust in psychologists or their big brothers in psychiatry. Mostly out of desperation and a paucity of ideas as to how to treat this pathetic man, I suggested EWOT. She was obviously underwhelmed with the idea and saw no relation to his condition and his oxygen supply. But being desperate and willing to "try anything" she agreed to the treatment. He was like putty and didn't care what you did to him or for him.

We put him on the stationary bicycle and virtually drove him to exercise for 15 minutes daily for a week and then anticipated cutting back to three times weekly if he showed any improvement. I really expected nothing and thought that surely he would have to be committed. Although it was not mentioned, it was obvious that she feared suicide.

On the morning of the third day after the commencement of treatment, she was astonished to find him in the kitchen at seven o'clock reading the morning paper. He pointed to the headlines and said: "Do you think this war will ever end?"

With tears in her eyes, she gently took the

paper away, embraced him and said: "I don't know, My Love, but I think *ours* has." For the first time since the tragedy, he wept.

When she told me the story, I almost cried myself.

Chapter 2

Oxygen and Your Body

Take a look at Figure 1 on page 24. Go ahead, I'll wait for you.

As you can see, you really don't have to start dying at 20. But most of us do. As the chart illustrates, by age 40 you have lost 20 percent of your oxygen-utilization ability and, by age 60, you have lost almost 40 percent of your ability to absorb and burn oxygen, your essential "fuel."

If you don't like charts, then just ignore them and trust me, but they do illustrate to those who are chart-friendly how crucial the oxygen-utilization issue is: If you don't absorb oxygen efficiently, you are going to age and die before your time. Who knows? If you follow this program with proper vigor, you might live long enough to see the fall of the Tower of Pisa or the end of the war in Yugoslavia, or even the birth of democracy in China. Nothing is guaranteed, of course.

The "gold standard" for measuring your body oxygen content is the level of oxygen in your arteries. Those are the vessels that leave your heart after they have been enriched with oxygen from your lungs. The vessels that you can feel pulsating from the pumping action of the heart are the arteries, like the one at your wrist the doctor feels to see if you are alive. The veins are the vessels that take the blood back to the heart and then to the lungs to be resupplied with oxygen. Those are the ones you see, but have no pulsation that you can feel. Parenthetically, it's the arteries, not the veins, that get plugged from eating too much sugar, vegetable fat, and smoking cigarettes.

Through the wonders of light technology, one can now take his blood oxygen level with a gadget attached to the ear. It's called an oximeter (ox-'im-ahter.) They are available from surgical supply houses. You may need a prescription to purchase this as well. Check the oximeter reading before and after EWOT and you will be delighted at the improved oxygen content of your blood.

A more detailed reading on your blood oxygen level can be obtained by getting it tested at a laboratory. If your doctor will cooperate you can do this, but I don't recommended it because of the cost, the time entailed, and the arterial puncture (not a vein, but a little artery deeper in the tissue than veins, and it hurts like the devil when stuck with a needle).

The measurement of the oxygen content of the arteries, indicated on your oximeter, is called the pO2. You will see this on the charts in this report. Don't worry about what it means except to remember that a normal pO2 is between 80 and 100. If you are down around 60, you have emphysema, cancer, or you have been hanging around the pool hall too much. If you are down to 40 then you are *really* in trouble because that is a normal value for your veins which have had over half the oxygen extracted for life-sustaining processes. You won't be walking around if you have a pO2 of 40.

But there is a definite down side on the oximeter, the "wonder of light technology" I mentioned. It is very expensive – a good one costs over $1,000! (Isn't it amazing how fast a doctor can spend your money?) The upside is that the test is unnecessary, like so many tests done in modern medicine. You don't need any testing at all. I have always been a pragmatist and have felt the patient was better off spending most of his money on treatment, not excessive testing. Such is the case here.

If you pink up, which you will, and you feel better, then you have accomplished your goal. If you insist on knowing your oxygen level every once in a while, go to a medical clinic or emergency room that administers the test. The test will cost you about $80, but that's better than spending $1,000.

A lot of people may complain of stress who are actually handling it very well. They may *think* they are suffering from stress, but if they have a pO2 of 80 to 100, don't feel sorry for them. They just like to whine a lot and probably enjoy their high stress position in life. Take away their stress and they would probably die of boredom; I know I would.

Most people, as they get older, don't handle stress as well, especially mental stress. That's when it's time to lighten up a little. Don't just *quit*, for heaven sakes, just relax enough to get your pO2 back up to 80, and EWOT can be lifesaving here. You would be amazed how quickly you can recover from life's little rabbit punches with a little EWOT.

Now let's look at how the aging process affects your oxygen level. The figures in the first chart on the next page (Figure 1, page 24), revealing the deterioration in your blood's ability to carry oxygen, are "normal" for our modern society. (It would be interesting to see what these values are in a stress-free society, if there is such a thing.) Figure I shows that, except for the period between ages 30 and 40, there is an average loss in oxygen-carrying capacity of the blood of about five points for every ten years of aging. (These are called millimeters of mercury, in case you are interested.)

Between 30 and 40, the drop is more dramatic and may be as high as 10 points, twice the drop in the other decades. That's why most professional athletes are in the history books after the age of 40. It's not because the younger players are better, because they're *not*. In fact, they aren't as good, because of a lack of experience. They just have more oxygen, which enhances their ability to perform.

As you can see from Figure 1, at age 80, if you are still with us, your pO2 is down to 68, close to the danger zone which starts at 60 points.

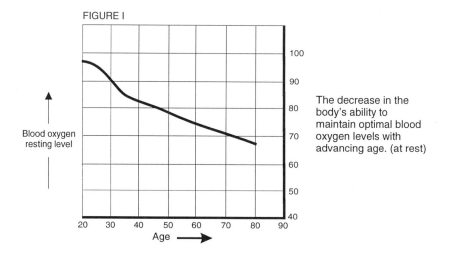

FIGURE I

The decrease in the body's ability to maintain optimal blood oxygen levels with advancing age. (at rest)

Figure II also reveals quite dramatically why the youngsters in sports push out the older guys, even the "immortals" who try to live on their reputation. Figure II demonstrates the ability to take

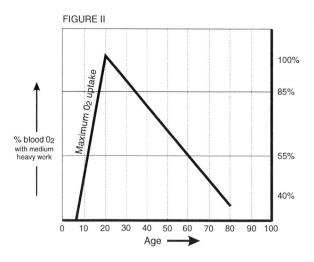

FIGURE II

The dramatic drop off in the body's ability to maintain a healthy blood oxygen level, when exercising, with advancing age.

up oxygen with a medium heavy work load. Between age 20 and 40 you have lost 20 percent of your ability to utilize oxygen with just *medium-heavy* work. You will never make it in the NFL or the NBA with those numbers. Better switch to golf.

Now let's look at an aspect of this remarkable therapy that you can "take to the bank," so to speak. *EWOT can have a profound effect on high blood pressure*, sometimes obviating the need for toxic, expensive, and questionably effective drugs. Even if only partially effective in lowering the pressure, this will enable you to take a smaller dose of medication that can make the difference between feeling well and wishing you were dead.

Table I (page 26) is an evaluation of 108 patients with a mean age of 68. You just wouldn't think patients at this relatively advanced age would respond to something as simple as exercise with oxygen but the improvement in their systolic (the upper number) blood pressure was impressive and probably extended their lives. Remember that "mean age" means that many of the participants in the experiment were much older than 68; one was 86.

The patients received 23 days of EWOT therapy. Their pO2 went up an average of 20 points. Their starting pO2 was an average of 67, a dangerously low value because, as you will recall, 60 points is where you enter the danger zone of heart failure, stroke, and a myriad of other often irreversible diseases. Whereas, 87 is a respectable pO2.

The changes in blood pressure were impressive enough that anyone with hyper-tension should add EWOT to their therapy program. The average drop in systolic pressure was 14 points. The improvement with some patients was considerably more. (And, as with every clinical experiment with humans, with some it was considerably less. Not everyone is going to benefit from *every* treatment. If that were so, doctors would be out of business.)

TABLE I

Factors measured ➤	Average Age	Duration of Therapy		Blood O2		Increase blood O2	Blood pressure		Blood pressure	
		total days	total days	before	after		Systolic before Rx	Diastolic before Rx	Systolic after Rx	Diastolic after Rx
				therapy						
Results	68	36	23	67	87	20	152	83	137	73
						*	△		□	

The effective lowering of blood pressure with EWOT. Blood oxygen increased by 20 points (*). Systolic blood pressure reduced from 152 (△) to 137 (□).

I never realized how many things can cause a stress reaction, as illustrated by the drop in blood pO2 values. Some of these findings are amazing and illustrate how we have been living in a sea of

20 percent oxygen — air — and never thought to try increasing it to treat stress.

Figure III demonstrates the remarkable stress placed on an individual in the "fast-paced executive" mode (Case A). This volunteer had his pO2 recorded before a prolonged business trip and then again on his return. He gave seven lectures, went to ten conferences, gave two interviews, went to two parties, and drove 1500 miles.

His pO2 before departure was 98, an excellent reading exhibiting good health. When he was retested on return from the trip he was, laboratory-wise, a basket case. His pO2 had plummeted to 82.

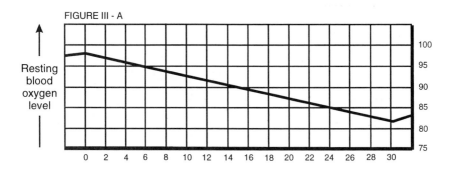

FIGURE III - A

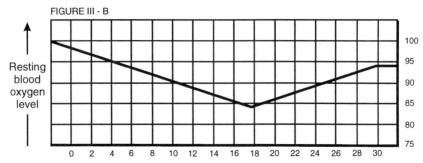

Travel and business stress and their impact with the blood oxygen levels.

Case B in this chart illustrates the same trauma to the body, but also demonstrates how a return to a "normal" life, even without EWOT, can cause regeneration of the body's oxygen-carrying capacity in a non-elderly person.

This volunteer traveled for 20 days, gave nine lectures, attended 11 conferences, gave nine interviews, went to nine parties, and flew from Berlin to Tokyo to Berlin. His initial pO2 was a perfect 100. On his return, it was 83. On the day of his return, he went back to his beloved gardening and, within five days had recovered to a respectable 94.

In the hotels where these high-powered executives stay when traveling, there is almost always a "fitness center." You can hardly call yourself a five-star hotel anymore without one of these exercise facilities. The hotels proudly promote them because they are in such great demand by travelers who know their lifestyle, while traveling, is not optimum. They just don't know how *un*-optimum it really is!

Immunizations

Those of you who have been reading **Second Opinion** or the works of the late Robert Mendelsohn will not be surprised at the effect of immunizations on the pO2 level. Figure IV makes it very clear that there is a powerful strain on the immune system, as evidenced by the incipient fall

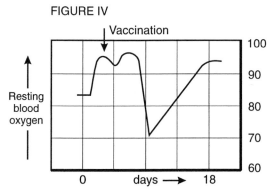

FIGURE IV

Vaccination gobbles up your blood oxygen, leaving you vulnerable to infection and other diseases.

in the pO2 *within minutes* of receiving the shot. This volunteer was a man of 64 who had a pO2 of 92 which is considered much higher than normal for his age. In less than two hours his pO2 had plummeted to 70 – a drop of over 20 percent in just 90 minutes.

Now what if this patient had suffered a heart attack an hour following the shot? This additional massive attack on his defenses would, in all probability, plunge his pO2 down below the 60 danger zone and he might die from "myocardial infarction." Acute hypoxemia (lack of oxygen) wouldn't even be considered in the diagnosis.

So if you are over 60 and are going to get a flu shot, not that I recommend them under any circumstances, you should get EWOT, bio-oxidative (hydrogen peroxide) therapy, or photoluminesence (or all three) before yielding to the magic needle.

In the smoking volunteer (figure V, page 31), *one cigarette* lowered the pO2 by ten points, from 95 to 85. Now that might not seem like a lot, but what if you do it *20 times a day*?

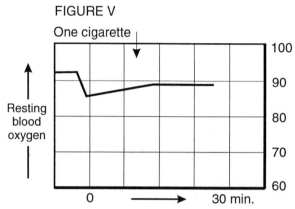

FIGURE V

The more you smoke, the lower your blood oxygen level will go.

Oxygen Killers

But the most punishing oxygen-suckers of all are major operations, cancer chemotherapy, X-ray therapy, and extensive burns. Figure VI (page 32) shows the instant effect that an operation has on the pO2.

Within 24 hours the pO2 drops below the danger zone *and it takes 50 days to make a reasonable recovery.* How many surgeons put their patients on EWOT following surgery? My guess would be none.

FIGURE VI

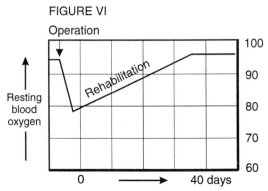

An operation is devastating to your ability
to carry sufficient oxygen in your blood.

Figure VII speaks for itself. The pO2 drops
steadily toward the danger zone as chemotherapy
continues and stays at or below 60 as long as
therapy continues.

FIGURE VII

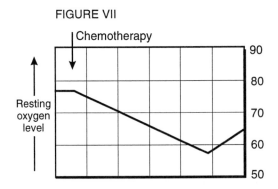

It is easy to see why EWOT is *vital*
during cancer chemotherapy. Few, if
any, receive it.

Remember that cancer *loves a low-oxygen environment* and so, although the drug may be killing some cancer cells, *it is encouraging the growth of more cancer* because of the low oxygen content of the tissues. Cancer hates oxygen, so it says, "thank you very much" and starts growing again, or a new type of cancer starts. Perhaps that's why in leukemia of children, the leukemia appears to have gone away after chemotherapy, but very often a new cancer, a lymphoma, develops and kills the child.

Because of the known fact that cancer hates oxygen, and cannot live in a high-oxygen environment, *I am convinced that EWOT is the best cancer preventive available at the present time.* As the effect is long-lasting, one treatment a month (assuming that you are healthy otherwise) should be enough to keep cancer away from your door. Unfortunately, no research has been done in this area, so I can't guarantee EWOT's effectiveness on cancer, but I'm still convinced that it will work as a preventive.

Other Oxygen Depressants

Even noise, in a healthy young volunteer,

depresses the pO2. After a rock concert, in a smoke-filled room, there's probably not enough oxygen among the kids to keep a debilitated sloth alive. God protects the young from their folly. Science hasn't figured out how, and never will.

One wonders how anyone could watch "Roseanne," "In Living Color," and "Beavis and Butthead," with the Grateful Dead playing in the background and come out of it alive. We live in an insane, degenerate world. You need all the oxygen you can get.

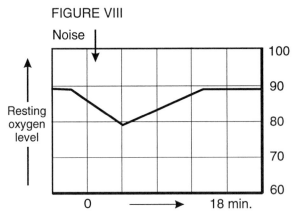

FIGURE VIII

A modern hazard that is hard to escape: noise-induced hypoxemia (low blood oxygen)

Severe physical exercise, such as marathon running, a prolonged boxing match, or lifting weights, strains even a healthy person. As Figure IX illustrates, there is a severe drop in the pO2 within three hours of starting the race and it stays down until the race is completed or the runner drops dead, which ever comes first. Most athletes engaging in extremely physically stressful sports do not live a long life.

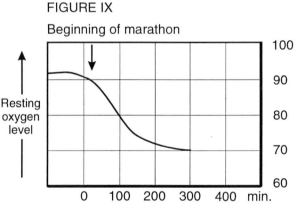

FIGURE IX

Beginning of marathon

A marathon is a terrible punishment to the body. Many die young.

The rehabilitative effect of EWOT is clearly shown by comparing the recovery of an influenza patient who recovered unaided by EWOT and one who received EWOT therapy. After 18 days, the EWOT-deprived patient *still* hadn't completely recovered, having less than an 80 pO2 (Figure X on the next page).

FIGURE X

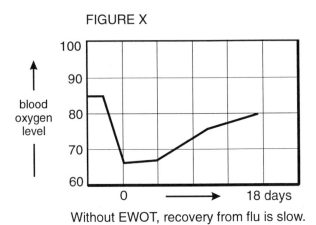

Without EWOT, recovery from flu is slow.

However, an influenza patient who was put on EWOT three days after his symptoms had cleared, had a normal pO2 of 95 within six days (Figure XI).

FIGURE XI

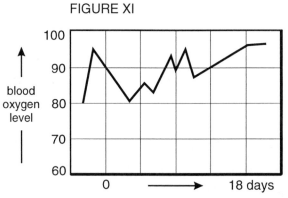

With EWOT, recovery from flu is dramatic.

One of the mysteries of EWOT is that once the blood oxygen level, as measured by the pO2, is brought up to a high normal level, say 90 or above, it will remain there until some other stressful event takes place. So you don't have to take EWOT every day for the rest of your life; just take it when needed. Science cannot explain why the oxygen level in the blood will remain high for *as long as a year* in some cases. Figure XII illustrates a case where the pO2 went from 75 to 93 in only two days and remained at that level for more than 52 weeks.

FIGURE XII

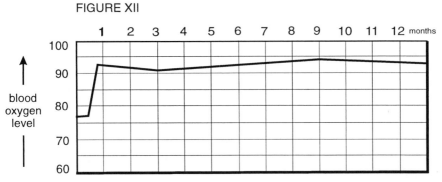

After EWOT, if there are no intervening traumas, excellent blood oxygen levels can often be maintained for over a year.

If you are 40, and your pO2 is 80, your doctor will probably say: "Your pO2 is within the normal range so you don't need extra oxygen." But if the optimal pO2 for children is 100, then why shouldn't *you* have the same advantage? Why should youth be wasted on the young? They don't handle it well. You may have a sonata, a poem, or a great novel to write. Don't grow old gracefully; fight it every way you can.

If you are 70, and your pO2 is also 70, which is considered "normal for your age" (see Figure 1), your doctor will tell you that's expected "at your age." So give up; there's nothing to be done about it.

Dr. von Ardenne answers this attitude with a statement (slightly annotated and emphasis added) that should be on the wall of every doctor's office and "anti-aging" clinic: "Until very recently, the decrease in pO2 with aging has been considered to be irreversible and, hence, *fatally governing the lifetime of man.* Experimenting upon myself, I discovered very unexpectedly that the pO2 decrease in old age *could be permanently re-elevated* to values of 100 by means of exercise with oxygen. *A value like this can be usually measured only in the juvenile.*" (See Figure XIII, page 39.)

FIGURE XIII

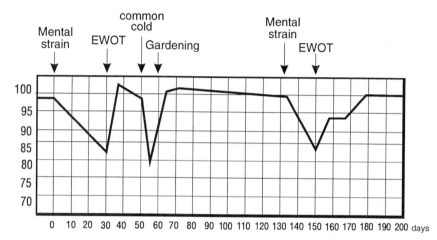

This 72-year-old volunteer illustrates dramatically the benefits of EWOT when under stress.

Now let's look at one more chart (Figure XIV, page 40) that summarizes life and its relationship to oxygen – when the oxygen stops, the party is over.

Note that the number at the far right of the bottom line, the "attained age," is 120 years. That's where your life should end on this earth if you are properly supplied with oxygen.

FIGURE XIV

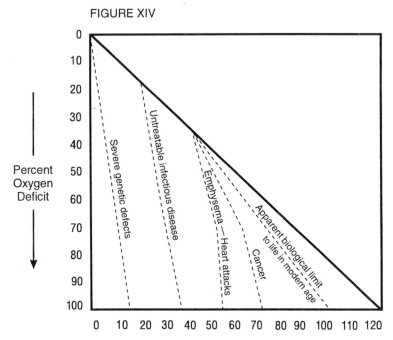

To extend *your* curve to the right - toward 120 - EWOT and other oxygenation therapies are essential during stress.

Chapter 3

Putting It Into Practice

There are an infinite variety of ways that you can take EWOT, so let's talk about some of the nuts and bolts about how to do it. If you are going to use a tread mill or a stationary bicycle, get a large tank of oxygen from the medical supply store (they're as heavy as your refrigerator). Your initial investment will be more, but the cost per treatment will be minimal. The tank can be refilled as needed; there's a gauge attached to tell you when to call the O2 man. The dealer will show you how to put on the little tube for nasal administration of the O2. It's quit simple and not at all uncomfortable. He can also show you how to turn on the oxygen and adjust the flow — it's easier than opening a bottle of "child-proof" aspirin.

Your only difficulty may be in getting the oxygen bottle for your treatment. In some states, you have to have a doctor's prescription for oxygen. If this is the case in your state, find a doctor who believes in natural therapies and ask him for the prescription. Surprisingly, there are a lot of wholistic doctors who are unaware of this therapy. Just take this monograph to him and he will probably become as enthusiastic as you are.

If you really want to look cool, and are physically fit, get a small bottle and wear it on your back, like a backpack, while you ride your bicycle around town. Or you can jog, do the polka, run with wolves, or whatever turns you on. Set the flow of oxygen to 6 litres per minute no matter what method you are using to get your oxygen.

Enjoyable Exercise

If you're 100 percent healthy, meaning your joints are all functioning, you don't have any heart disease, everything is on go — then your best bet is the stationary bicycle. Remember, we're not trying to set any speed records. Start at two miles per hour (your speed is registered on your speedometer). It's a good idea, unless you're an accomplished athlete, to wear a pulse monitor (available at "fitness"-type stores) on your ear. If your pulse gets over 130, slow down. Naturally, if you feel faint, stop and rest. Use common sense. If you are not sure just how fit you are and you are a little nervous, just go for two or three minutes at a slow speed the first time and find your level of tolerance.

Now if you are a little old and run down, like my editor, then don't use the bicycle. Settle for something less strenuous, like light or medium-heavy bar bells. You can even do it in bed and work up from there. Your results are naturally going to be slower, but if you persist, you might become the oldest winner of the Tour de France bike race.

You'll want to work up to about 15 minutes on the stationary bicycle. Wear a head set and play music, or whatever you're interested in, on your Walkman. You'll be surprised how long 15 minutes is when you're having to actually work. Set a timer and don't look at the clock because, if you do, the 15 minutes will seem like 15 hours. Until you are acclimated, it's best to have someone around, like a doctor or a nurse.

The "golden triangle" for a long life, assuming that you are doing everything else right (We can't negate *all* of your bad habits), consists of EWOT, bio-oxidation, and photoluminescence. If that doesn't get you to age 100 or beyond, then you chose the wrong parents; we can't do anything about that — and neither can EWOT!

I strongly recommend that you employ this simple and effective modality if you are over 20 years of age — healthy or not. If you are young and healthy, it will delay the aging process. If you are young and sickly, it may help your illness. If you are over the age of 50, no matter what your state of health, I emphatically recommend EWOT.

Ref: M. von Ardenne, *Stress* journal, Volume 2, 1981.

H. Selye, *The Stress of Life*, New York: McGraw-Hill, 1964.

Index

Get a *Second Opinion* every month with Dr. Douglass' medical newsletter

Here's a shocker for you: Did you know that cancer, heart disease, the common cold, and a host of other "incurable" or "chronic" illnesses, are in many cases now completely reversible?

Did you know that garlic can help with certain forms of depression? That cabbage juice can cure the most stubborn, painful ulcer — almost immediately? That extra magnesium in your diet can reduce tendencies toward anxiety, obesity, and even heart palpitations?

It's true. And it's exactly the kind of helpful medicine that can help keep you out of your doctor's office. It'll help you live longer, feel better, even look younger. You can only find such invaluable advice in *Second Opinion*.

With *Second Opinion,* you'll see your doctor less ... spend a lot less money ... and be much happier and healthier while you're at it. Go ahead and subscribe today! When you do, we'll give you one of the reports or books described in the next two pages absolutely free ... you choose the one you want!

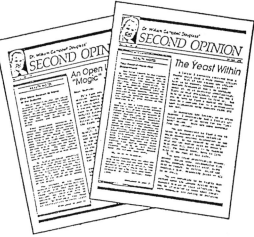

Choose your free book/report on the next three pages!

Don't drink your milk!

If you knew what we know about milk ... BLEEECHT! All that pasteurization, homogenization and processing is not only cooking all the nutrients right out of your favorite drink. It's also adding toxic levels of vitamin D.

This fascinating book tells the whole story about milk. How it once was nature's nearly perfect food ... how "raw," unprocessed milk can heal and boost your immune system ... why you can't buy it legally in this country anymore, and what we could do to change that.

Dr. Douglass travelled all over the world, tasting all kinds of milk from all kinds of cows, poring over dusty research books in ancient libraries far from home, to write this light-hearted but scientifically sound book. And if you like, it's yours free when you subscribe to *Second Opinion!*

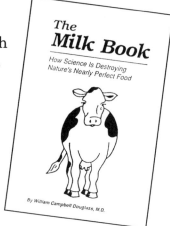

You've got more to choose from!
See the next two pages.

Is it possible this generations-old treatment could actually
STOP AIDS, CANCER, TUBERCULOSIS
and other killer diseases of our time?

We've seen this procedure save lives every place it has been used, from Russia to Central Africa to the practices of a handful of physicians in this country farsighted enough to use it.

What is it? It's called "photo-luminescence." It's a thoroughly tested, proven therapy that's been miraculously successful, with absolutely no dangerous side effects.

This remarkable treatment works its incredible cures by stimulating the body's own immune responses. That's why it cures so many ailments — and why it's been especially effective against AIDS!

Yet, 50 years ago, it virtually disappeared from the halls of medicine. Why has this incredible cure — proven effective against many ailments, from AIDS to cancer, influenza to allergies, and so much more — been ignored by the medical authorities of this country?

That's why Dr. Douglass wrote **Into the Light**. This hard-hitting, fully documented book tells the success story of photo-luminescence — what it can heal, who it's helped, who covered it up and why.

Get **Into the Light** now and discover the whole story for yourself.

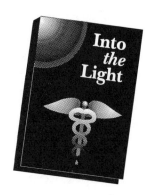

You've got more to choose from!
See the next page.

Choose one of our special reports as your free gift!

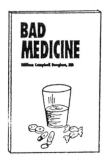

AIDS: Why It's Much Worse Than They're Telling Us, And How To Protect Yourself And Your Loved Ones

Yes, AIDS is easy to catch. No, it isn't limited to just a few groups of society. People who've never engaged in questionable behavior or come within miles of an infected needle are contracting this deadly scourge. To protect yourself, you must know the truth.

Dangerous (Legal) Drugs

If you knew what we know about the most popular prescription and over-the-counter drugs, you'd be sick. That's why Dr. Douglass wrote **Dangerous (Legal) Drugs**. He gives you the low-down on 15 different categories of drugs: everything from painkillers and cold remedies to tranquilizers and powerful cancer drugs.

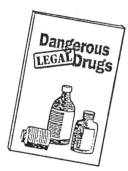

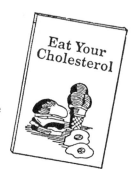

Bad Medicine

Do you really need that new prescription or that overnight stay in the hospital? In this report, Dr. Douglass reveals the common medical practices and misconceptions endangering your health. Best of all, he tells you the pointed (but very revealing!) questions your doctor prays you never ask!

Eat Your Cholesterol

Never feel guilty about what you eat again! Dr. Douglass shows you why red meat, eggs, and dairy products aren't the dietary demons we're told they are. But beware: This scientifically sound report goes against all the "common wisdom" about the foods you should eat. Read with an open mind!

To subscribe and choose your free gift, please use the order form on the next page.

ORDER HERE

I'd like to buy the following:

Qty.	Title	Price	Amount
____	1 Year/*Second Opinion*	$49*	$_____
____	The Milk Book	$14.95	$_____
____	Into the Light	$15.95	$_____
____	AIDS: What They're Not Telling You	$ 8.95	$_____
____	Dangerous (Legal) Drugs	$ 8.95	$_____
____	Bad Medicine	$ 8.95	$_____
____	Eat Your Cholesterol	$ 8.95	$_____
	If not subscribing, add shipping/handling per order: $2.50 first item, 50¢ each additional item		$_____
		TOTAL	$_____

❑ My payment of $_____ is enclosed.
   (*Foreign subscribers add $13 per year.)
❑ Charge my: ❑ MasterCard ❑ Visa

Card#_____

Signature_____ Exp._____

NAME _____

ADDRESS_____

CITY_____STATE_____ZIP_____

TELEPHONE_____

EWOT94

Call Toll-Free
1-800-728-2288
Fax: 404-399-0815

Mail to: *Second Opinion*
P.O. Box 467939 • Atlanta, GA 31146-7939

"Love Second Opinion!"

Here are just a few good things we've heard about Dr. William Campbell Douglass and *Second Opinion.*

You are indeed a "second opinion." You are brilliant and provocative.

Your *Second Opinion* is a breath of fresh air. Keep up the good work, and for God's sake, continue bowing to no one.

I am glad to find someone, especially an actual medical doctor, who is saying what I have suspected for some time.

Frankly, I trust your judgment. I base many of the questions I ask my family physician on information I get from your superb newsletter.

William Campbell Douglass, MD graduated from the University of Rochester, the Miami School of Medicine, and the Naval School of Aviation and Space Medicine. He has been named the National Health Federation's "Doctor of the Year."

Dr. Douglass is a popular speaker who has appeared on radio and television hundreds of times over the years. The author of five books and numerous articles, he also travels widely. A former practicing physician who in the past operated clinics on three continents, Dr. Douglass is now editor-in-chief of the alternative medicine newsletter *Second Opinion.*

ORDER HERE

I'd like to buy the following:

Qty.	Title	Price	Amount
____	1 Year/*Second Opinion*	$49*	$_____
____	The Milk Book	$14.95	$_____
____	Into the Light	$15.95	$_____
____	AIDS: What They're Not Telling You	$ 8.95	$_____
____	Dangerous (Legal) Drugs	$ 8.95	$_____
____	Bad Medicine	$ 8.95	$_____
____	Eat Your Cholesterol	$ 8.95	$_____

If not subscribing, add shipping/handling per order:
$2.50 first item, 50¢ each additional item $_____

TOTAL $_____

☐ My payment of $_____ is enclosed.
  (*Foreign subscribers add $13 per year.)
☐ Charge my: ☐ MasterCard ☐ Visa

Card#_____

Signature_____ Exp._____

NAME _____

ADDRESS_____

CITY_____STATE_____ZIP_____

TELEPHONE_____

EWOT94

Call Toll-Free

1-800-728-2288

Fax: 404-399-0815

Mail to: *Second Opinion*
P.O. Box 467939 • Atlanta, GA 31146-7939

"Love Second Opinion!"

— G.B.F., Mt. Pleasant, TX

Here are just a few good things we've heard about Dr. William Campbell Douglass and *Second Opinion*.

You are indeed a "second opinion." You are brilliant and provocative.

— Dr. T.M.D., Leonia, NJ

Your *Second Opinion* is a breath of fresh air. Keep up the good work, and for God's sake, continue bowing to no one.

— R.V.F., Ph.D., Santa Barbara, CA

I am glad to find someone, especially an actual medical doctor, who is saying what I have suspected for some time.

— W.M.M., Ashland, VA

Frankly, I trust your judgment. I base many of the questions I ask my family physician on information I get from your superb newsletter.

— J.M., Jacksonville, FL

William Campbell Douglass, MD graduated from the University of Rochester, the Miami School of Medicine, and the Naval School of Aviation and Space Medicine. He has been named the National Health Federation's "Doctor of the Year."

Dr. Douglass is a popular speaker who has appeared on radio and television hundreds of times over the years. The author of five books and numerous articles, he also travels widely. A former practicing physician who in the past operated clinics on three continents, Dr. Douglass is now editor-in-chief of the alternative medicine newsletter *Second Opinion*.